50 Paleo Pizza Recipes

Your Pizza Cravings Satisfied … The Paleo Way!

I0412763

Disclaimer

What This Book is All About

Craving pizza on a strict diet? Don't want to break your record of a few successful days of no-carb diet but can't stop dreaming about the cheesy goodness of your favorite meal? What if you can enjoy your favorite food and still maintain your diet? This book is perfect for you. You can satisfy your pizza needs with these Paleo pizza recipes.

A Paleo diet is a healthy way of staying fit. This diet ensures you eat a nutritional meal which helps you in staying energetic, strong and healthy. Paleo diet is filled with refined food and helps prevent degenerative diseases like depression, cancer, obesity, infertility, heart diseases and more.

This book contains 50 Paleo pizza recipes which anyone can easily make, as well as:

a) Details about Paleo Diet
b) List of Paleo food items
c) Paleo pizza crust recipe

Some of these recipes contain pizza dough making directions as well. While the rest of the topping recipes can be used with the pizza crust recipe mentioned in the starting of this book.

Let's start making some delicious healthy pizzas!

Contents

Introduction

Paleo is the short form of Paleolithic. The Paleo diet has started gaining popularity through media and books. This diet is based on the concept that in order to remain fit, people should start consuming whole, real and unprocessed foods. These foods are healthy, fresh and beneficial for our bodies. This diet can also be called as 'Ancestral,' 'Nutrient-Dense,' 'Whole Food,' 'Grain-Free,' or 'Primal'. With its gradual popularity, more and more individuals are getting aware about the significance of eating healthy food.

Here is a short version list of what to eat and what not to eat on a Paleo diet:

What to Eat

a) Seeds
b) Nuts
c) Eggs
d) Fresh Vegetables
e) Fresh fruits
f) Fish/seafood
g) Grass-produced meats
h) Oils (coconut, avocado, macadamia, flaxseed, walnut, olive)

What Not to Eat

a) Candy / Junk / Processed Food
b) Cereal grains
c) Refined vegetable oils
d) Salt
e) Processed foods
f) Potatoes
g) Refined sugar
h) Dairy
i) Legumes (including peanuts)

Paleo Food List

Meats

1. Lamb Rack
2. Chicken Wings
3. Chicken Leg
4. Chicken Thigh
5. Chicken Breast
6. Turkey
7. Grass Fed Beef
8. Ground Beef
9. Pork
10. Pork Tenderloin
11. Pork Chops
12. Steak
13. Bacon
14. Poultry
15. Bison
16. Shrimp
17. Veal
18. New York Steak
19. Buffalo
20. Lobster
21. Venison
22. Steaks
23. Salmon
24. Clams
25. Rattlesnake
26. Chuck Steak
27. Quail
28. Lean Veal
29. Pheasant
30. Ostrich
31. Bison Steaks
32. Turtle
33. Reindeer
34. Wild Boar
35. Eggs (duck, chicken or goose)
36. Bison Jerky
37. Beef Jerky
38. Bison Ribeye
39. Bison Sirloin
40. Bear
41. Lamb Chops
42. Kangaroo
43. Rabbit
44. Goose
45. Emu
46. Elk
47. Goat

Sea Food

1. Lobster
2. Halibut
3. Scallops
4. Clams
5. Shrimp
6. Oysters
7. Crayfish
8. Salmon
9. Mackerel
10. Trout
11. Bass
12. Walleye
13. Crawfish
14. Swordfish
15. Sardines
16. Tuna
17. Red Snapper
18. Shark
19. Sunfish
20. Crab
21. Tilapia

Fruits

1. Plums
2. Pineapple
3. Watermelon
4. Persimmon
5. Tangerine
6. Pears
7. Strawberries
8. Peaches
9. Star Fruit
10. Passion Fruit

11. Rhubarb
12. Papaya
13. Raspberries
14. Orange
15. Pomegranate
16. Nectarine
17. Mango
18. Cherries
19. Lychee
20. Cherimoya
21. Lime
22. Melon
23. Cassava
24. Lemon
25. Carambola

26. Kiwi
27. Cantaloupe
28. Honeydew melon
29. Boysenberries
30. Guava Blueberries
31. Blackberries
32. Grapes
33. Grapefruit
34. Banana
35. Gooseberries
36. Avocado
37. Apricot
38. Cranberries
39. Apple
40. Figs

Vegetables

1. Artichoke
2. Mushrooms
3. Asparagus
4. Mustard Greens
5. Beet Greens
6. Onions
7. Beets
8. Parsley
9. Bell Peppers
10. Parsnip
11. Broccoli
12. Peppers (all kinds)
13. Brussels Sprouts
14. Pumpkin
15. Cabbage
16. Purslane
17. Carrots
18. Radish
19. Cauliflower
20. Rutabaga

21. Celery
22. Seaweed
23. Collards
24. Spinach
25. Cucumber
26. Squash (all kinds)
27. Dandelion
28. Swiss Chard
29. Eggplant
30. Tomatillos
31. Endive
32. Tomato
33. Green Onions
34. Turnip Greens
35. Kale
36. Turnips
37. Kohlrabi
38. Watercress
39. Lettuce

Nuts and Seeds

1. Almonds
2. Pine Nuts
3. Brazil Nuts
4. Pistachios (unsalted)
5. Cashews
6. Pumpkin Seeds
7. Chestnuts

8. Sesame Seeds
9. Hazelnuts
10. Sunflower Seeds
11. Macadamia Nuts
12. Walnuts
13. Pecans

Oils

1. Coconut Oil
2. Olive Oil
3. Macadamia Oil
4. Avocado Oil
5. Grass fed Butter

Preparing Paleo Pizza Crust

Ingredients

Olive oil – ½ cup

Water – ½ cup

Celtic sea salt – ½ tsp

Tapioca flour – 1½ cups

Diced garlic – 1 tsp

Egg – 1

Italian seasoning – 1 tsp

Almond flour – 2 tbsp

Directions

1. Pour olive oil in a small pan. Add garlic, seas salt and water.
2. Bring the mixture to a boil.
3. Remove the pan from heat and add tapioca flour.
4. Mix well and leave it for 8 minutes. Include egg and Italian seasoning in the dough.
5. Flatten the dough out on parchment paper.
6. Keep the thickness around ¼" to ½" to get a crispy pizza crust. If you keep the dough thicker than this, your crust will turn out soft.
7. On the top of your dough, sprinkle almond flour (1tsp). Flip the dough and sprinkle the rest of almond flour on this side as well.
8. Place the pizza dough on a stainless steel sheet and out it in the oven after removing parchment paper's top piece.
9. Bake for 25 minutes at 350 ºF.
10. Once the crust is done, you can add your choice of topping and bake at 350 ºF for 10 minutes more.

Preparing Paleo Pizza/Tomato Sauce

Ingredients

Tomato paste – 6 oz

Tomatoes – ½ cup (crushed)

Dried oregano – ½ tsp

Dried basil – ½ tsp

Dried parsley – ½ tsp

Onion flakes – ½ tsp (minced)

Onion powder – ½ tsp

Garlic powder – ½ tsp

Salt and pepper – to taste

Directions

1. Mix all these ingredients in a sauce pan.
2. Simmer for 10 minutes, stirring a few times.
3. Pour in a bowl.
4. Delicious tomato/pizza sauce ready for the pizza crust.

50 Paleo Pizza Recipes

Paleo Pizza Bites

Ingredients

Large pepperoni – 20 -30 pieces (5-7 oz)

Pizza sauce

Black olives – as needed

Bell peppers – 1

Mushrooms – as needed

Green onions – 1

Directions

1. Heat your oven to 400 °F.
2. Put the pepperoni slices in a baking sheet and put them in oven for 8 minutes or until they are crisp.
3. While the pepperoni slices are in the oven, start preparing the topping. Cut all bell peppers, green onions, black olives and mushrooms in to small pieces.
4. Take out the pepperoni slices from the oven when they are done and spread pizza sauce on them.
5. Top it with the rest of the ingredients.
6. Place the pizza bites in a baking sheet and place it in the oven for 10 minutes.

Layered Casserole Pie Pizza

Ingredients

For Top Layer:

Pepperoni or Salami - 16 slices

For Sauce and Meat Layer:

Ground Beef – 1 lb

Tomato Sauce – 1 cup

Italian seasoning – 1 tbsp

Garlic powder – ½ tsp

Sea salt – ¼ tsp

Oregano – ½ tsp

For Veggie Crust Layer:

Raw zucchini – ½ medium sized (ground or grated)

Raw cauliflower – 1 cup (ground or grated)

Garlic cloves – 2

Eggs – 2 (beaten)

Coconut floor – 3 tbsp

Coconut oil – 1 tbsp

Salt – ¼ tsp

Directions

1. Grease casserole dish and put oven on preheat at 400 °F.
2. In a fry pan, cook ground beef until brown. Remove excess grease.
3. Add sea salt, oregano, garlic powder, Italian seasoning and tomato sauce.
4. Stir the mixture on medium heat until it starts bubbling. Cover the pan and lower the heat. Let it cook for 6 minutes.
5. Add, in a food processor, garlic cloves, cauliflower and zucchini. Process these ingredients until they look similar to rice granules. Or you can also grate these vegetables.
6. Combine the garlic cloves, cauliflower and zucchini mixture with coconut flour, sea salt, coconut oil and eggs. Mix well till it becomes a paste like dough. Break up clumps and cover.
7. Take the ground beef off from the stove after stirring it. Start spreading this mixture into the bottom of casserole dish.
8. Spoon the veggie paste dough over the meat layer. Spread it evenly in a smooth layer over the meat.
9. On the top, place salami or pepperoni slices and put the dish in the oven.
10. Bake for 30 minutes or until the top layer starts looking brown and crispy.

Crusty Cauliflower Pizza

Ingredients

Cauliflower – 1 (medium)

Kosher salt – ¼ tsp

Dried basil – ½ tsp

Dried oregano – ½ tsp

Garlic powder – ½ tsp

Egg – 1

Pizza sauce – as needed

Bell pepper – 2

Onions – 2

Directions

1. Put oven on preheat at 450 ºF. Place parchment paper on pizza pan and spray it with cooking oil.
2. Take the cauliflower, wash it and let it dry. Cut the florets and put them in a food processor to process for 30 seconds. You will get a powdery form of mixture. Put it in a bowl and cover.
3. Microwave the cauliflower for 4 minutes and place it on a clean towel. Allow it to cool.
4. Once it is cooled, wrap the towel and squeeze it. Wring it multiple times to remove all excess water.
5. Put the cauliflower in a clean bowl. Start adding kosher salt, garlic powder, dried oregano, and dried basil and mix well.
6. Add egg in the mixture and mix.
7. Start forming dough into a crust with your hands into the parchment paper you oiled earlier. Make sure you tap it down nicely and tightly.
8. Don't make the dough too thick or too thin.
9. Place the pizza pan in the oven and bake for 11 minutes or till it starts turning golden brown.
10. Remove from the oven and start adding the toppings.
11. Spread the sauce evenly on the crust; place sliced bell peppers and onions. You can include more veggies if you want.
12. Put the pizza back in the oven for 5-7 minutes.
13. Let it cool for a few seconds and serve.

Arugula and Prosciutto Pizza

Ingredients

Egg – 1

Roma tomato – 1 (sliced thinly)

Dried basil – 1 tsp

Dried oregano – 1 tsp

Olive oil – 1 tsp

Eggplant – 1 (grated)

Arugula – ½ cup

Prosciutto – ¼ lb

Almond meal – ¼ cup

Flax seed meal – ¼ cup

Pepper and salt – 1 tsp or to taste

Directions

1. Put oven on preheat at 350 °F.
2. In a clean towel, place the grated eggplant. Wrap the towel and squeeze to remove any excess liquid. Transfer into a bowl.
3. Add almond meal, flax meal, pepper and salt. Mix all ingredients well.
4. Transfer the mixture into a baking sheet and spread it with hands into 1/8 inch layer.
5. Put the baking sheet into the oven and bake for 35 minutes. Remove from oven and place a lightly oil parchment paper over the crust.
6. Flip the crust and peel off the parchment paper from the bottom carefully. Brush lightly with oil and place this side up in the oven for 15 minutes.
7. Remove from oven and place Roma tomatoes, dried basil, dried oregano, arugula and prosciutto on the top of the crust.
8. Bake for 10 minutes more and serve.

No Cheese Paleo Pizza

Ingredients

No Cheese Sauce:

Raw cashews – ½ cup

Raw pine nuts – ¼ cup

Sea salt – 1 tsp

Dried oregano – ½ tsp

Basil – ½ tsp

Ground black pepper – 1/8 tsp

Garlic powder – a pinch

Nutritional yeast – 1 tsp (optional)

Unsweetened almond milk – 1½ cup

Lemon juice – 2 tbsp

Vinegar – 1 tbsp

Gelatin – 8 tsp

Olive oil – ¼ cup

Topping:

Pizza sauce – 1 ½ cup

Ripe tomato – 1 large (sliced)

Fresh basil – 15 leaves

Dried oregano – ½ tsp

Directions

No Cheese Sauce:

1. In a saucepan, place nuts and cover them with water. Put on high heat and bring to a boil.
2. Lower the heat to medium and bring to a light boil for 15 minutes or till nets are soft.
3. Drain the water and put the nuts in a food processor.
4. Add yeast, garlic powder, black pepper, basil and salt in the food processor and blend till a paste is formed.
5. In a saucepan, put olive oil, gelatin, vinegar, lemon juice and almond milk. Cook on high heat and bring to a boil. Lower the heat to medium and bring the mixture to a light boil for 5 minutes all the while stirring continuously.
6. Transfer this mixture in food processor and process till it becomes smooth.
7. Grease lightly the ramekins and pour the mixture into them. Place them in the fridge for 2 hours or till the mixture firms.

Assembling the Pizza:

1. Preheat your oven at 375 °F. Place the dough (see pizza crust recipe at the start of the book) into pizza pan. The thickness must not be more than ¼". Bake for 25 minutes.
2. Remove the no cheese sauce from fridge and cut in thin slices or cubes. Set aside.
3. Take out the pizza crust and spread pizza sauce on top of it.
4. Top with basil leaves, no cheese sauce slices, and a dash or dried oregano.
5. Bake the pizza for 5-8 minutes or until the no cheese sauce starts to melt. Serve.

Cauliflower Olive and Ground Beef Pizza

Ingredients

For Sauce:

Diced tomato – 1 can (small)

Onion – 1 (finely chopped)

Garlic – 2 cloves (chopped)

Salt – ½ tsp

Black pepper – ½ tsp

Oregano – 1 tbsp

Onion powder – 1 tsp

Garlic powder – 1 tsp

Fennel seeds – ¼ tsp (coarsely ground)

Chili peppers – to taste (crushed)

Ground clove – to taste

Ground cinnamon – to taste

Honey – 1 tsp (optional)

For Garnish:

Mushrooms – 3-4 (sliced)

Red bell pepper – ¼ (diced)

Ground beef – 150 g (cooked)

Onion powder – ½ tsp

Garlic powder – ½ tsp

Sea salt – to taste

Black pepper – ¼ tsp

Green olives – 4 tbsp (sliced)

Fresh basil – few leaves

Directions

Sauce:
1. In a sauce pan, add garlic, onion, oregano, chili peppers, fennel seeds, garlic powder, salt, black pepper, cinnamon and clove. Cook for 2-3 minutes on medium heat till onions turn translucent.
2. In the mixture, add honey (optional) and canned tomatoes and bring to a boil. Let it simmer on low heat for 15 to 20 minutes. The water will evaporate and the sauce will thicken.

Crust:
1. To make the crust, follow the Paleo Pizza Crust recipe given in the start of this book.

Topping:
1. Spread tomato sauce on the crust as much as you desire.
2. Top with ground beef, bell peppers and olives.
3. Put the pizza in the oven and bake for 10 minutes or till the edge of the crust starts to color.
4. After it is done, let it cool for 2 minutes, sprinkle fresh basil and serve.

Zucchini Pizza

Ingredients

Zucchini – 2 large (sliced)

Tomato – 1 (sliced)

Green bell pepper – 1 (sliced)

Tomato sauce – 2 cups

Olive oil – 2 tbsp

Sea salt – to taste

Black pepper – to taste

Fresh basil – few leaves

Crushed red chili – to taste

Directions

1. Put oven on preheat at 380°F. Cover a pizza pan with parchment paper and sprinkle with olive oil.
2. Follow the Paleo pizza crust recipe and put the pizza in the oven for 25 minutes.
3. Top the crust with tomato sauce and place zucchini slices, tomato slices and bell pepper slices on top.
4. Sprinkle with a little olive oil, crushed red chili, black pepper and salt.
5. Place the pizza in the oven for 10 minutes and then let it cool for 2 minutes.
6. Sprinkle with fresh basil leaves and serve.

Supreme Meatza

Ingredients

Ground beef – 1 lb

Mix Italian herb – 1 tsp

Garlic powder – ¼ tsp

Onion powder – ¼ tsp

Salt – ¼ tsp

Black pepper – ¼ tsp

Tomato sauce – 1 can

Pepperoni – to taste (sliced)

Bell pepper – 1 (diced)

Red onion – 1 (thinly sliced)

Black olives – to taste (sliced)

Mushrooms – to taste (sliced)

Directions

1. Put your oven on preheat at 450°F.
2. Mix onion powder, garlic powder, pepper, salt and ground beef in a bowl.
3. Sprinkle a little olive oil on parchment paper and place it in pizza pans. Divide the mixture in two pans evenly. Spread it and pat it down smoothly.
4. Afterwards, spread tomato sauce over the crust. Top it will mushroom, pepperoni slices, onions, bell peppers and olives.
5. Place the pizza in oven and bake for 25 minutes or till it is done.
6. Cool for 2 minutes and serve.

Feasty Meaty Pizza

Ingredients

Crust:

Cauliflower – 1 medium

Eggs – 3

Thyme – 1 tsp

Oregano – 1 tsp

Basil – 1 tsp

Parsley – 1 tsp

Almonds – 1 cup (finely ground)

Flax seeds – 1/3 cup

Topping:

Tomato paste – 3 tbsp

White onions – ¼ (cut in strips)

Streaky bacon – 2 rashers (cut in chunks)

Cooked turkey – 1 slice (cut in pieces)

Pepperoni – 3 slices (cut in pieces)

Directions

Crust:

1. Preheat oven at 450 °F.
2. In a food processor, grind cauliflower till it reaches consistency of rice granules.
3. In a bowl, whisk eggs. Add flax seeds, almonds, parsley, oregano and thyme. Include cauliflower and mix well.
4. Pour the mixture into a pizza pan and ensure the thickness is not more than ¼".
5. Put in the oven to bake for 15 minutes.

Topping:

1. Once the crust is done, spread tomato sauce on it.
2. Add onions, bacon, turkey and pepperoni on top.
3. Return it in oven and bake for 10 minutes then serve.

Primal Paleo Pizza

Ingredients

Water – 1 cup

Coconut flour – ½ cup

Coconut oil – ½ cup

Roasted tomatoes – ¼ cup (pureed)

Sea salt – 1 tsp

Ground beef – 1 lb (seasoned)

Granulated garlic – 1tsp

Thyme – 1 tsp

Tapioca flour – 1 ½ cups

Oregano – 1 tsp

Eggs – 2

Fresh basil – few leaves

Directions

1. Put oven on preheat at 350 °F.
2. Mix coconut oil, salt and water in a sauce pan and bring to a boil.
3. Remove the pan from heat. Add tapioca flour and garlic. Mix well and leave it for 5 minutes.
4. Include eggs and mix well. Add in coconut flour.
5. Start kneading the dough till it becomes smooth.
6. Sprinkle a little olive oil on parchment paper and place it on pizza pan.
7. Spread the dough on a pizza pan with your hands and spread it evenly.
8. Put the pan in an oven for 30 minutes or till it starts turning brown. The underside will be golden brown.
9. Take out the crust and thinly spread roasted tomato puree on it.
10. Top with thyme, oregano and ground beef.
11. Put the pan back in the oven for 10 minutes.
12. Let it cool and serve.

Paleo Taco-licious Pizza

Ingredients

Portabella mushroom caps – 4 (large)

Ground beef – 1 lb

Taco seasoning – 2 tbsp

Water – ½ cup

Taco sauce – ¼ cup

Lettuce – ½ (diced)

Tomato – 1 (diced)

Onion – 1 (diced)

Directions

1. Put your oven on preheat at 400 °F.
2. Brushing mushrooms with oil on both sides, season them with pepper and salt.
3. In a baking sheet (foiled lined), place all the mushrooms with stem side up.
4. Bake for 8-10 minutes. Flip them and bake for another 5 minutes.
5. Using a skillet, cook the ground beef over medium heat till it is brown.
6. Add water and taco seasoning. Mix the mixture well till it thickens and the meat is well cooked.
7. When the mushrooms are done, pour taco sauce on the stems of every mushroom.
8. Add ¼ of seasoned ground beef on each mushroom. Top them with onion, tomato and lettuce.
9. Put them back in the oven and bake for 5 minutes.

Margherita Pizza

Ingredients

Crust:

Almond flour – 2 cups

Arrowroot flour – ½ cup

Gluten-free baking powder – 2 tsp

Salt – 1 tsp

Black pepper – 1 tsp

Dried oregano – 2 tsp

Dried basil – 1 tsp

Dried marjoram – 1 tsp

Garlic powder – 1 tsp

Onion powder – 1 tsp

Coconut oil – ¼ cup

Eggs – 2

Sauce:

Roasted tomatoes – 1½ cup (crushed)

Tomato paste – ½ cup

Garlic – 1 clove

Onion – 2 tbsp (finely minced)

Dried oregano – 1 tsp

Dried basil – 1 tsp

Pepper and salt – to taste

Topping:

Tomato – 1 medium (thinly sliced)

Basil – 10 leaves

Directions

1. Put the oven on preheat at 325 °F.
2. Add eggs, coconut oil, onion powder, garlic powder, marjoram, basil, oregano, black pepper, salt, baking powder, arrowroot flour and almond flour in a mixing bowl.
3. Stir the mixture until dough is formed.
4. Roll dough into a ball and spread evenly in a pizza pan lined with parchment paper.
5. Put in oven and bake for 20-25 minutes or till the crust gets firm.
6. In a sauce pan, add tomato paste and roasted tomatoes and cook on medium heat.
7. Add pepper, salt, basil, oregano, minced onion and garlic.
8. Stir well and let it simmer for a while.
9. Once the crust is done, spread the sauce all over the crust.
10. If you want a soft pizza, add a thick layer of sauce but if you want a crisp pizza, the layer of sauce must be thin.
11. Add basil and tomato topping and put the pizza back in the oven.
12. Bake for another 20 minutes, let it cool and serve.

Simple Paleo Pizza

Ingredients

Tomato sauce – 2 cups

Oregano – ½ tsp

Onion – 1 (sliced)

Olives – ½ cup

Basil – 10 leaves

Bell pepper – 1 (sliced)

Zucchini – ½ (sliced)

Directions

1. Preheat oven at 400 °F. Place a parchment paper on pizza pan and drizzle with olive oil.
2. Follow the Paleo Pizza Crust recipe (mentioned in the start on the book) and make the pizza crust.
3. Once the crust is done, remove from oven and let it cool for 5 minutes.
4. Evenly spread a thin layer of tomato sauce on the crust.
5. Add oregano, onions, bell peppers and zucchini on top. Sprinkle with olives and basil leaves.
6. Return it to the oven and bake for another 10 minutes.

Rosti Paleo Pizza

Ingredients

Tomato sauce – 2 cups

Oregano – ½ tsp

Lettuce – ½ (diced)

Carrots – 2 (sliced)

Cauliflower – ½

Green Onions – 1 (diced)

Tomato – 1 (sliced)

Cucumber – 1 (sliced)

Onions – 1 (sliced)

Bell Peppers – 1 (sliced)

Mushrooms – ½ cup

Cabbage – ½ (diced)

Salt and pepper – to taste

Red chili flakes – to taste

Directions

1. Make the pizza crust by following the Paleo Pizza Crust recipe (mentioned in the start on the book).
2. Once the crust is done, add all the toppings.
3. Add mushrooms, cabbage, bell peppers, onions, cucumber, tomato, green onions, cauliflower, carrots and lettuce.
4. Sprinkle oregano, red chili flakes, salt and pepper on top.
5. Return the pizza back in the oven and bake for 10 minutes more.
6. Let it cool for 2 minutes and serve.

Marinara Paleo Pizza

Ingredients

<u>For Crust:</u>

Cauliflower – 1 small (cut in florets)

Egg – 1 (slightly beaten)

Sea salt – ½ tsp

Oregano – ½ tsp

Black pepper – to taste

Garlic – ½ tsp (diced)

Thyme – ½ tsp

<u>Topping:</u>

Tomato sauce – 1 cup

Green olives – 3 tbsp (sliced)

Black olives – 3 tbsp (sliced)

Capers – 1 tbsp

Oregano – 1 tbsp

Grilled chicken – ½ cup (diced)

Olive oil – as required

Directions

1. Put oven on preheat at 450 °F. Sprinkle olive oil on parchment paper and place it in pizza pan.
2. Process cauliflower in a food processor and put it in a bowl. Microwave it for 8 minutes.
3. Place cauliflower in a clean towel and squeeze out the moisture.
4. Put the cauliflower in a bowl and add pepper, salt, oregano, garlic, thyme and egg. Mix well till dough is formed and knead it with hands.
5. Spread the dough on the pizza pan with thickness not more than ¼".
6. Bake the crust in the oven for 20 minutes or till slightly golden.
7. Take out the crust and let it cool for 2 minutes.
8. Pour the tomato sauce and spread evenly on the crust. Add capers, olives and grilled chicken on top. Sprinkle with oregano and lightly drizzle with olive oil.
9. Put it back in the oven and back for another 10 minutes.
10. Serve hot.

Paleo Pesto Chicken Pizza

Ingredients

Pesto sauce:

Basil leaves – 2 cups

Pine nuts – ½ cup

Garlic – 2 cloves

Olive oil – ½ cup

Salt – to taste

Crust:

Cauliflower – 3 cups (chopped)

Eggs – 3

Almond meal – 2 cups

Garlic powder – ½ tsp

Onion flakes – ½ tsp

Salt and pepper – to taste

Topping:

Cooked chicken – 1 cup (shredded)

Onion – 1 (sliced and sautéed)

Broccoli – ½ cup (diced)

Tomato – 1 (sliced and sun dried)

Basil – 12 leaves

Directions

Pesto sauce:

1. Blend garlic, pine nuts and basil leaves in a food processor.
2. Add salt, pour in olive oil and blend again till a smooth mixture is formed.

Crust:

1. Put oven on preheat at 450 °F. Drizzle olive oil on parchment paper and put in pizza pan.
2. Blend cauliflower in a food processor till it reaches the consistency of rice granules.
3. Mix cauliflower, pepper, salt, onion flakes, garlic powder, almond meal and eggs in a bowl till dough is formed.
4. Spread this dough on the pizza pan and bake for 15 minutes.

Topping:

1. Take out the crust from the oven and spread the pesto sauce on it.
2. Top it with tomatoes, broccoli, onions and chicken. Sprinkle basil leaves on it and bake for 10 minutes.
3. Serve warm.

Fritza

Ingredients

Ground beef – 1 ½ cup (cooked and diced)

Red pepper – ½ cup (diced)

Green pepper – ½ cup (diced)

Onion – ½ cup (finely diced)

Mushrooms – 1 cup (sliced)

Tomato – 1 cup (chopped)

Olives – ¼ cup (diced)

Eggs – 10 (beaten and seasoned with garlic powder, basil and oregano)

Milk – ½ cup

Directions

1. Preheat oven to 400 °F.
2. Sauté onions and peppers in an oven proof skillet for a few minutes or till soft.
3. Add mushrooms and sauté for 2 minutes then add ground beef and tomatoes.
4. Cook for 1 minute more. Pour in the egg mixture all over the skillet.
5. Let it cook for a few minutes on medium heat till the edges start turning brown.
6. Put the skillet in to the oven and bake for 5-10 minutes or till the eggs are set.
7. Take out of the oven and sprinkle olives, oregano and basil on top.
8. Serve hot.

Salmon Paleo Pizza

Ingredients

Smoked salmon – ½ cup (sliced)

Tomato puree – 1 cup

Capers – ½ cup

Olives – ½ cup

Directions

1. Follow the Paleo Pizza Crust recipe (mentioned in the start on the book) to make the pizza crust.
2. Once the crust is done, spread the tomato puree evenly on the crust.
3. Top with smoked salmon, capers and olives.
4. Place in the oven again and bake for 10 minutes.
5. Serve hot.

Veggie Low Carb Pizza

Ingredients

Sweet Italian peppers – 1 cup (chopped)

Olive oil – 1 tsp

Onions – 2 (chopped)

Italian seasoning – 1 tsp

Oregano – 1 tsp

Almond meal – 2 cups

Salt and pepper – to taste

Eggs – 2 (or egg whites – 4)

Kale – 1 cup (chopped)

Mushrooms – 5 (sliced)

Shallot – 1 (finely chopped)

Tomatoes – 1 cup (diced)

Garlic – 1 tsp (crushed)

Basil – 10 leaves

Directions

1. Preheat your oven to 400 °F. Cover a cake pan with parchment paper sprinkled with olive oil.
2. In a skillet, add Italian peppers, onions, oregano, salt and pepper. Sauté them till they become soft and set aside.
3. In another skillet, add olive oil, kale, shallot, garlic, Italian seasoning, salt and pepper. Sauté these as well till they soften and turn bright green. Take off from stove.
4. To make the crust, add almond meal and eggs in a mixing bowl. Mix well.
5. Start molding this crust in the cake pan. Put it in the oven for 15-20 minutes or till it start turning brown. (Keep checking the crust as it may turn brown really quickly)
6. Once the crust is done, start layering the toppings.
7. Add mushrooms, then a layer of sauté peppers, followed by kale mixture, layer of tomatoes and sprinkle with basil leaves.
   Put it in the oven for about 10 minutes and serve.

Chicken Tikka Paleo Pizza

Ingredients

<u>Cashew Cream:</u>

Raw Cashews – 1 cup

Water – 4 cups

<u>Topping:</u>

Chicken – 1 lb (boneless and skinless)

Tomato sauce or strained tomatoes – 2 cups

Yellow onion – ½ (chopped)

Garlic – 2 cloves (minced)

Garam masala powder (You can purchase this from an Indian grocery store) – 2½ tbsp

Dried ginger – 1 tsp

Paprika – ½ tsp

Salt – 1 tsp

Cayenne pepper – to taste

Cashew cream – ½ cup

Fresh cilantro – ½ cup (chopped)

Directions

1. In a cooker, add cayenne pepper, salt, paprika, ginger, garam masala, garlic, onions and tomato sauce. Add chicken at the top and cook on low heat for about 6 hours.
2. When 30 minutes are left for your sauce to cook, preheat your oven at 350 °F.
3. Make the crust by following the Paleo Pizza Crust recipe (mentioned in the start on the book).
4. To make the cashew cream, Heat 3 cups of water. Soak the raw cashews in the water for 25-30 minutes. Drain the cashews and blend it with ¾ cup water. Stop when the mixture becomes smooth and thick. If it is too thick, add water to reach your desired consistency.
5. Remove the sauce from the heat. Take out the chicken from the sauce and chop it roughly.
6. Add cashew cream in the sauce and add the chopped chicken as well.
7. When the crust is done, sprinkle on olive oil and spread the chicken and sauce mixture on the crust.
8. Place the pizza back in the oven and bake for 10-15 minutes.
9. Take out from oven and sprinkle the top with fresh cilantro.
10. Start serving while warm.

Pizza Paleo Style

Ingredients

Coconut floor – ½ cup

Almond meal – 1 cup

Baking powder – 1 tsp

Garlic powder – 2 tsp

Eggs – 4

Olive oil – 3 tbsp

Coconut milk – ½ cup

Beef – 1 lb (chopped and seared)

Mushroom – 1 cup (sliced)

Bell peppers (yellow and green) – 1 cup (sliced)

Pizza sauce – 1 cup

Directions

1. Put oven on preheat at 375 °F.
2. Mix garlic powder, baking powder, almond meal, coconut flour in a bowl, mix well and sift.
3. Start adding slowly coconut milk, eggs and olive oil while slowly stirring continuously.
4. Dough will start to form. Knead it and place it on a greased pizza pan. The dough must be spread evenly and smoothly all over the pan.
5. Place it in the oven and bake for 20 minutes.
6. Take it out from the oven and start spreading the pizza sauce on the crust.
7. Top it with beef, mushrooms and bell peppers.
8. Return to the oven and bake it for another 10 minutes.

Portobello Primal Pizza

Ingredients

Portobello mushroom caps – 2

Tomato sauce – ¼ cup

Oregano – 1 tsp

Olive oil – 2 tbsp

Green peppers – 1 cup (sliced)

Red onions – 1 cup (sliced)

Chicken – 1 lb (seared and chopped)

Directions

1. Put oven on preheat at 375 °F.
2. In an iron pan, heat olive oil.
3. Add mushrooms and let them cook for 10 minutes, flipping once.
4. Top the mushrooms with sauce, chicken, onions and green peppers.
5. Sprinkle oregano on top and a little olive oil as well.
6. Put the iron pan inside an oven and bake for 20 minutes or till the veggies are done.

Pesto Paleo Pizza

Ingredients

Pesto paleo sauce:

Basil leaves – 2 cups

Pine nuts – ½ cup

Garlic – 3 cloves (minced)

Olive oil – ½ cup

Kosher salt – ½ tsp

Red pepper flakes – to taste

Topping:

Roasted tomatoes – 1 can

Pesto paleo sauce – 1 cup

Chicken sausage – 1 lb (chopped)

Mushrooms – 1 cup (sliced)

Shallot – 1 (sliced)

Basil – 1 tsp

Directions

1. Preheat your oven at 400 °F.
2. To make the presto sauce, combine all the ingredients in a blender and blend well. Transfer it in a bowl and set aside.
3. To make the crust, follow the Paleo Pizza Crust recipe (mentioned in the start on the book).
4. Cook the chopped chicken sausages till they turn light brown.
5. In another pan, sauté the shallot along with basil and mushrooms on medium heat, till they become soft.
6. Once the crust is done, spread the pesto paleo sauce evenly all over it. Place roasted tomatoes on top along with chicken sausage, mushrooms and shallot.
7. Bake for 10 minutes and serve.

Hawaiian Thin Crust Paleo Pizza

Ingredients

<u>For crust:</u>

Eggs – 4

Coconut floor – ¼ cup

Yogurt – ¼ cup

Oregano – 1 tsp

Sea salt – to taste

<u>Topping:</u>

Tomato paste – 1 cup

Onion – ¼ (finely sliced)

Garlic – 2 cloves (minced)

Pineapple chunks – ½ cup

Ham – 2 oz (shredded)

Directions

1. Preheat oven at 400 °F.
2. Mix yogurt, salt and eggs. Whisk together well.
3. Sift in coconut floor and stir the mixture till it thickens. Add oregano.
4. Pour the mixture on a lined pizza pan and put it in the oven.
5. Bake for 10 minutes.
6. Mix garlic and tomato paste together and spread it on the crust evenly once it is baked.
7. Top it with ham, onions and pineapples.
8. Put the pizza pan back in the oven and bake for 10 minutes more.
9. Serve warm.

Pizza Flatbread
Ingredients

Raw sunflower seed flour – ½ cup	Dried basil – 1 tsp
Tapioca flour – ½ cup	Dried oregano – 1 tsp
Egg – 1	Tomato sauce – 1 cup
Olive oil – 2 tbsp	Bell peppers – 2 (sliced)
Water – 1 tbsp	Onion – 1 (sliced)
Salt – to taste	Pepperoni – ½ cup (sliced)
Garlic powder – 1 tsp	Olives – ½ cup (sliced)

Directions

1. Preheat oven to 350 °F. Place parchment paper on pizza pan and sprinkle with olive oil.
2. In a bowl, add sunflower seed flour, tapioca flour, egg, water, olive oil, garlic powder and salt. Mix well.
3. Add dried basil and oregano. Stir it till it becomes like a thick paste.
4. Spread the mixture in pizza pan evenly. The layer must be thin.
5. Bake for 15 minutes.
6. Take out and top it with tomato sauce, bell peppers, onion, pepperoni and olives.
7. Return it in the oven and bake for another 5-10 minutes till the topping is done.

Paleo Meaty-zza

Ingredients

<u>Crust:</u>

Italian sausage – 2 lb (minced)

Eggs – 2

<u>Topping:</u>

Pizza sauce – 1 cup

Oregano – 1 tsp

Red pepper flakes – to taste

Bell pepper – 1 (sliced)

Onion – 1 (sliced)

Zucchini – 1 (sliced)

Olives – 1 (sliced)

Broccoli – 1 (sliced)

Mushrooms – 1 (sliced)

Directions

1. Preheat oven at 375 °F.
2. Combine the minced sausage and eggs using your hands.
3. When it is mixed well, spread it in an iron skillet or baking dish drizzled with olive oil.
4. Put the dish in the oven and bake for 25 minutes or till it starts to pull away from the sides.
5. Once the crust is done, remove from the oven.
6. Top it with pizza sauce, bell pepper, onion zucchini broccoli and mushrooms, Sprinkle with olives, oregano and red pepper flakes.
7. Place it in the oven and bake for 10 minutes or till it begins to brown.

Bacon Cauliflower Pizza

Ingredients

Tomato sauce – 1 cup

Cauliflower head – 1

Egg whites – 2

Coconut floor – 1 cup

Onion – 1

Spinach – ¾ cup

Bacon strips – ½ cup

Garlic powder – ½ tsp

Oregano – 1 tsp

Thyme – 1 tsp

Basil – 1 tsp

Black pepper – 1 tsp (crushed)

Directions

1. Put oven on preheat at 400 °F.
2. Blend cauliflower head till it reaches rice granules consistency.
3. Put cauliflower in a pan and steam till it softens. Set aside.
4. Cook beef strips and shred them in small pieces.
5. Warm up the tomato sauce.
6. Once the cauliflower has cooled down, add all the spices, coconut flour and egg whites. Mix well.
7. Place this mixture on a pizza pan and spread it evenly. Place the pizza pan in the oven and bake for 15 minutes.
8. Take out from oven and spread the sauce on it. Top it with spinach, bacon, onion, bell pepper. Sprinkle with basil.
9. Return in the oven and bake for 10 minutes.

Mini Pizzas
Ingredients

Crust:

Coconut flour – 4 tbsp

Eggs – 4

Coconut milk – ¼ cup

Oregano – 1 tsp

Basil – 1 tsp

Sea salt – 1 tsp

Topping:

Tomato paste – 2 tbsp

Red onion – ¼ (chopped)

Garlic – 2 cloves (finely chopped)

Olive oil – 1 tbsp

Directions

Crust:

1. Mix all herbs, milk and eggs in a bowl.
2. Slowly pour coconut flour and stir continuously to make a thick paste.
3. Sprinkle the baking tray with olive oil and spoon 1 tsp of batter on the tray. Make tiny circles within 2-3" distance of each other.
4. Put the tray in the oven (preheated at 400 °F). Let them bake for 10 minutes.

Topping:

1. In a pan, fry garlic and red onions on low heat for 10 minutes.
2. Once the mini pizza crusts are done spread the tomato sauce on all of them.
3. Top them with garlic and red onion mix, sprinkle oregano, ground black pepper and basil on top.
4. Put the tray back in the oven and bake for 10 minutes.

Paleo Casserole Pizza

Ingredients

Eggplant – 1 (sliced)

Italian sausage – ¾ lb (cooked and chopped)

Mariana sauce – 1 cup

Coconut oil – 1 tbsp

Thyme – 1tbsp

Basil – 1 tsp

Red pepper flakes – 1 tsp

Oregano – 1 tsp

Directions

1. Preheat oven at 350 °F.
2. Sprinkle pan with coconut oil, and cover it with eggplant. Make sure to make only one even layer of eggplant.
3. Spread Marinara sauce on the eggplant and top it with ½ tsp each of thyme, basil, oregano and red pepper flakes.
4. Add the Italian sausages and spread another layer of marinara sauce over it.
5. Sprinkle with ½ tsp each of thyme, basil, oregano and red pepper flakes.
6. Put the pan in the oven for an hour.
7. Let it cool for 2 minutes and serve.

Caramelized Onions and Honey Bacon Pizza

Ingredients

Grape tomatoes – 1 pint

Olive oil – 1 tbsp

Bacon slices – 4

Onion – 1 (thinly sliced)

Ground black pepper – 1 tsp

Honey – 1 cup

Directions

1. Make the crust by following the Paleo Pizza Crust recipe (mentioned in the start on the book).
2. In a bowl, add olive oil and toss in grape tomatoes.
3. Transfer the grape tomatoes into a broiler placed with parchment paper. Let it broil for 5 minutes or till grape tomatoes become soft. Set them aside.
4. In a pan, cook bacon on medium heat till it becomes crisp. Place the bacon on a clean towel and dry it.
5. Discard the bacon grease from the pan but leave almost 2 tbsp of it. On high heat, cook onions for 10 minutes or till they soften. Transfer on the towel with the bacon.
6. When the crust is prepared, spread the grape tomatoes on it. Add the onions evenly and sprinkle the bacon across the pan. Drizzle little ground pepper on top.
7. Place the pan in the oven and bake for 12 minutes.
8. Transfer on a cutting board and drizzle some honey over the pizza.
9. Serve warm.

Best Paleo Pizza
Ingredients

Coconut flour – 1½ cup

Psyllium Husk powder – 5 tbsp

Baking sode – 2 tsp

Sea salt – 1 tsp

Egg whites – 8

Boiling water – 1 cup

Garlic – 3 cloves

Oregano – 1 tsp

Basil – 1 tsp

Onion – 1 (sliced)

Tomato sauce – 1 cup

Green peppers – 3-4 (sliced)

Olives – ½ cup

Grilled chicken – 1 lb (chopped)

Directions

1. Preheat oven at 350 °F.
2. Mix sea salt, basil, oregano, baking powder, psyllium husk powder and coconut flour in a glass bowl.
3. Pour in the egg whites and mix well till a thick paste is formed.
4. Pour in boiling water. Mix till dough becomes firm.
5. Place parchment paper on pizza pan and drizzle with olive oil.
6. Spread the dough in the pan and place it in the oven to bake for 1 hour.
7. Once the crust is done, spread the tomato sauce evenly.
8. Top with all the veggies and chicken. Sprinkle oregano and basil on top.
9. Put in the oven for 5 minutes.

Paleo Pizza Pie

Ingredients

Italian sausage – 1 lb (minced)

Bell pepper – 1 (chopped)

Onion – 1 (chopped)

Mushrooms – 1 cup (chopped)

Red pepper flakes – ¼ tsp

Garlic powder – 2 tsp

Dried basil – 2 tsp

Oregano – 1 tsp

Tomato sauce – 1 cup

Almond flour – ½ cup

Baking powder – ½ tsp

Eggs – 6

Salt – ½ tsp

Mushrooms – 1 cup (sliced)

Olives – ½ cup

Pepperoni – 1 cup (sliced)

Cooked bacon – 1 cup (chopped)

Directions

1. Preheat oven at 450 °F. Sprinkle olive oil on an oven dish.
2. In a large frying pan, fry Italian sausages. With a potato masher, mash the sausages in small pieces. Add red pepper flakes, mushrooms, bell peppers and onions. Cook for 12 minutes on medium heat. Lower the heat and add tomatoes, oregano, basil, salt and garlic. Mix well and remove from heat.
3. Prepare the crust in a medium bowl by adding almond flour, baking powder, salt and eggs. Combine this mixture and pour in the oven dish.
4. Add veggie and sausage mix over the crust. Top it with olives, bacon and pepperoni.
5. Sprinkle a little oregano, red pepper flakes and basil on top and put the dish in the oven.
6. Bake for 20 minutes. Let it sit for 10 minutes and serve.

Crusty Coconut Flour Paleo Pizza

Ingredients

Eggs – 4

Greek yogurt – ¼ cup

Coconut flour – ¼ cup

Italian seasoning – ½ tsp

Salt – to taste

Garlic powder – ½ tsp

Bell pepper – 1 (sliced)

Onion – 1 (sliced)

Olives – ½ cup

Pepper flakes – to taste

Oregano – to taste

Directions

1. In a bowl, mix Greek yogurt and eggs.
2. Add in coconut flour and Italian seasoning. Mix till there are no lumps.
3. Spread the mixture on a parchment paper covered pan as thinly as you can.
4. Sprinkle with salt and garlic powder.
5. Bake in the oven for 12 minutes.
6. Take out and spread pizza sauce on it.
7. Add bell peppers, onions and olives.
8. Sprinkle with oregano and red pepper flakes.
9. Return in the oven and bake for 10 minutes.
10. Serve while hot.

Easy-Peasy Paleo Pizza

Ingredients

Cauliflower head – 1 (grated)

Yogurt – ½ cup

Salt – 1 tsp

Basil – 1 tsp

Oregano – ½ tsp

Garlic powder – ½ tsp

Eggs – 2

Directions

1. In a bowl, add grated cauliflower, eggs, garlic powder, oregano, basil, salt and yogurt. Mix well.
2. Spread it evenly on a parchment lined pan.
3. Bake for 50 minutes on 400°F.
4. Once done, take out from the oven and spread tomato sauce over it.
5. Top up with mushrooms, green coriander and onions.
6. Put the pizza back in the oven and bake for another 10 minutes.

Pizza Zucchini Boat

Ingredients

Zucchinis – 2 large

Grilled chicken – 1 lb

Zucchini pulp – 1 cup

Curry powder – ¼ tsp

Thyme – ½ tsp

Pizza sauce – 1 cup

Black olives – ½ cup

Onion – 1 (sliced)

Tomato – 1 (sliced)

Directions

1. Put your oven on preheat at 400°F.
2. Lengthwise cut the 2 zucchini and scoop the insides out leaving only the skin.
3. In a bowl, place the pulp. Add grilled chicken, tomato sauce, curry powder, thyme, onion, black olives and tomatoes.
4. Mix the ingredients and scoop them over the zucchini skins.
5. Bake for 25 minutes and serve.

Stuffed Chicken Pizza

Ingredients

Chicken breasts – 4 large

Garlic powder – ¼ tsp

Mushrooms – 3 (diced)

White onion – 1/3 cup (diced)

Sun-dried tomatoes – 3 (diced)

Pepperoni – 32 slices

Fresh basil – 6 leaves (sliced)

Bread crumbs – 1 cup

Pizza sauce – 1 cup

Almond flour – 1/8 cup

Dried basil – ½ tsp

Dried oregano – ½ tsp

Black olives – ½ cup (sliced)

Salt and pepper – to taste

Directions

1. Put your oven on preheat at 450°F.
2. In a pan, sauté sun-dried tomatoes, onions and mushrooms on medium high heat for 5 minutes or till veggies are tender. Remove from stove.
3. Leave one side connected and fillet the chicken. Unfold them and pound them to ½ inch thickness.
4. Place the tomatoes, onions and mushrooms sauce on one side of the chicken and pour pizza sauce over it.
5. Top it with pepperoni slices and fresh basil. Folding the chicken piece, cover the mixture inside.
6. If needed, secure with a tooth pick. Repeat this process on all chicken breasts.
7. In a separate bowl, add salt, oregano, basil, bread crumbs and almond flour. Mix the ingredients.
8. Take one chicken breast and dip one side in the crumbs mixture. Top with olives. Place this chicken breast, crumb side up, on a foiled covered baking sheet. Repeat this process with the remaining chicken breasts.
9. Place the baking sheet in the oven and bake for 25 minutes.
10. Serve hot.

Portobello Pizzas

Ingredients

Portobello mushrooms – 4

Sausage – 1 (cooked)

Bell pepper – 1 (chopped)

Onion – 1 (chopped)

Tomato – (chopped)

Pizza sauce – 1 cup

Salt and pepper – to taste

Oregano – ½ tsp

Thyme – ½ tsp

Directions

1. Put your oven on preheat at 375°F.
2. After removing stems of mushrooms, bake them for 5 minutes on a baking pan drizzled with olive oil.
3. Remove from the oven. Spread pizza sauce on top.
4. Add all the chopped veggies and sprinkle with oregano and thyme.
5. Place the baking sheet back in the oven and bake for 20 minutes.
6. Serve hot.

Meatza Mexicana
Ingredients

Crust:

Ground beef – 1 lb

Chili powder – 2 tsp

Cumin – ½ tsp

Paprika – ½ tsp

Salt – ½ tsp

Garlic – 2 cloves (crushed)

Topping:

Tomato sauce – 1 cup

Green bell pepper – 1 (thinly sliced)

Red onion – 1 (thinly sliced)

Avocado – ½ cup (diced)

Fresh cilantro – 1 tbsp (chopped)

Directions

1. Put your oven on preheat at 400°F.
2. Mix together chili powder, cumin, paprika, salt, garlic and ground beef.
3. Separate half of the meat and roll in a ball. Spread the meat evenly in a pie pan. Smooth out the meat till it has even thickness.
4. Repeat this process with the other half of the meat.
5. Put both pie pans in the oven and bake for 15 minutes or till the edges of the meat start turning brown and it is cooked through.
6. Take out the pans and let them cool.
7. Place the meat crusts on a baking sheet lined with parchment paper. Spread the tomato sauce all over the meat crusts. Top with onions and bell peppers.
8. Place the backing sheet in the oven and bake for 15 minutes.
9. Remove from the oven and sprinkle with avocado and fresh cilantro.

Pizza Paleo Margherita

Ingredients

Chicken – 1 lb (diced)

Sun-dried tomatoes – ½ cup (crushed)

Dried oregano – ½ tsp

Basil – ½ tsp

Salt and pepper – to taste

Mushrooms – ½ cup (sliced)

Olives – ½ cup

Artichoke – ½ cup

Directions

1. Prepare crustcrust by following the Paleo Pizza Crust recipe (mentioned in the start of the book).
2. Once the crust is done, spread it with tomato sauce.
3. Add on chicken, tomatoes, pepper, basil, salt and oregano.
4. Top with sautéed mushrooms, artichokes and olive. Sprinkle basil and oregano on top.
5. Place it in the oven for 15 minutes or until golden.

Frittata Fajita

Ingredients

Grilled chicken – 1 lb

Red onion – 1 (diced)

Bell pepper – 1 (finely chopped)

Olive oil – 1 tbsp

Green onions – 1 (sliced)

Cilantro – ½ (chopped)

Tomato sauce – ½ cup

Eggs – 6-8

Salt – to taste

Directions

1. Put your oven on preheat at 375°F.
2. In a non-stick pan, pour olive oil and n medium high heat sauté bell pepper and red onion. Add chicken and let it cook for a while till it starts getting brown.
3. Include tomato sauce, cilantro and green onions. Stir a little and remove form stove.
4. In a bowl, whisk the eggs and salt. Add this mixture over the veggie and chicken mixture.
5. Put on slow heat and stir till ¼ eggs are cooked.
6. Put the pan in oven and bake for 10 minutes or till the eggs are cooked through.
7. Cut slices and serve.

Salad Paleo Pizza

Ingredients

Pepperoni slices – 30 (chopped)

Green bell pepper – 1 (sliced)

Yellow bell pepper – 1 (sliced)

Eggplant – 1 (diced)

Red onion – 1 (diced)

Mushrooms – ½ cup (sliced)

Red chili flakes – to taste

Olive oil – 2 tbsp

Black olives and Green olives – ½ cup (chopped)

Banana peppers – ½ cup (chopped)

Fresh basil – 4-5 leaves

Tomato sauce – 1 cup

Directions

1. Sauté pepperoni slices till they are crispy. Set aside to dry.
2. Add olive oil in a pan and mushrooms, eggplant, onions and peppers. Sauté these ingredients for 3-4 minutes.
3. Prepare crustcrust by following the Paleo Pizza Crust recipe (mentioned in the start of the book).
4. When the crust is done, spread tomato sauce evenly and thinly over it.
5. Add pepperoni slices. Top with veggie mixture.
6. Sprinkle with banana peppers, olives, basil and red chili flakes.
7. Palace the crust back in the oven and bake for 10 minutes.

Bacon Lovers Pizza
Ingredients

Bacon – 6 strips

Eggs – 3

Tomato sauce – 1 cup

Broccoli – ½ cup (chopped)

Jalapeño peppers – 3 (sliced)

Red onion – 1 (sliced)

Argula – ½ cup (chopped)

Directions

1. Put your oven on preheat at 400°F.
2. Place bacon in a baking dish and bake till golden and crispy.
3. In a bowl, whisk 3 eggs together and pour over bacon strips.
4. Return the dish in the oven and bake for 3-4 minutes or till the mixture is firmed.
5. Take out the dish from the oven and drain any grease left in the dish.
6. Spread tomato sauce over it. Add broccoli, jalapeño peppers, red onions and argula on top.
7. Place the dish back in the oven and bake for 10 minutes.

Paleo Chicken Fajita Pizza

Ingredients

Chicken breasts – 1 lb (cooked and chopped)

Red bell pepper – 1 (chopped)

Green onions – 2 (chopped)

Cilantro – 2 tbsp (chopped)

Lime juice – 2 tbsp

Salt and pepper – to taste

Tomato sauce – 1 cup

Directions

1. In a bowl, mix together tomato sauce, salt, pepper, cilantro and lime juice.
2. Add chopped chicken in the mixture and stir.
3. Prepare crust by following the Paleo Pizza Crust recipe (mentioned in the start of the book).
4. Once the crust is done, spread this mixture all over it evenly.
5. Top with green onion and bell pepper. Sprinkle some red chili flakes if you want.
6. Put the crust in the oven and bake for 10-15 minutes.

Puttanesca Roasted Pepper Pizza

Ingredients

Ground beef – 1 lb (cooked and chopped)

Tomatoes – ½ cup (crushed)

Dried oregano – ½ tsp

Basil – ½ tsp

Salt and pepper – to taste

Olive oil – 2 tbsp

Red pepper flakes – to taste

Garlic clove – 1 (chopped)

Anchovies – 6

Capers – 1 tbsp

Olives – ½ cup

Roasted peppers – ½ cup (chopped)

Directions

1. Prepare crust by following the Paleo Pizza Crust recipe (mentioned in the start on the book).
2. Pour olive oil in a bowl and sauté tomatoes, red pepper flakes, garlic clove, roasted peppers, anchovies, salt and pepper.
3. Add ground beef and stir.
4. Take out the crust when it is done and spread the ground beef mixture all over the crust.
5. Top with capers, olives, basil, dried oregano and red pepper flakes.
6. Return to the oven and bake for 5-10 minutes.

Casserole Breakfast Pizza

Ingredients

Chicken steak – 1 lb (cooked and chopped)

Eggs – 8

Bell pepper – 1 (sliced)

Green chilies – 1 cup (diced)

Onion – 1 (sliced)

Directions

1. Put your oven on preheat at 400°F.
2. In a bowl, mix together green chilies, bell pepper, onion and chopped chicken.
3. Pour this mixture in a baking dish and bake for 20 minutes or till eggs are set.
4. Serve hot.

Meatball Pizza
Ingredients

Olive oil – 2 tbsp

Tomato sauce – ½ cup

Basil – ½ tsp

Green bell pepper – 1 (sliced)

Ground beef – 1lb

Egg – 1

Garlic powder – 1tsp

Paprika – 1tsp

Salt and pepper - to taste

Onion – ½ small (minced)

Spinach – 1Tbsp

Parsley – 1Tbsp

Directions

1. Put your oven on preheat at 375°F.
2. In a bowl, mix together egg, beef, garlic powder, paprika, salt and pepper, onion, spinach and parsley.
3. Scoop equal portions of this mixture with the help of an ice cream scoop (you can use your hands as well).
4. Place them on a baking sheet lined with parchment paper.
5. Place this baking sheet in the oven and bake for 3-5 minutes. Flip them and bake for another 3-5 minutes (it is perfectly fine if they are not done properly as they will be baked again with the pizza). Take out of the oven and set aside.
6. Prepare crust by following the Paleo Pizza Crust recipe (mentioned in the start of the book).
7. Spread tomato sauce on the baked crust. Add meatballs and green bell pepper. Sprinkle basil on top.
8. Bake for 10-15 minutes and serve hot.

Zucchini Pepperoni Baked Pizza

Ingredients

Zucchini – 3 medium

Tomato sauce – 1 cup

Italian seasoning – 1 tsp

Garlic powder – 1 tsp

Salt and pepper – to taste

Turkey pepperoni – 12 slices

Water – ¼ cup

Directions

1. Put your oven on preheat at 425°F and sprinkle a baking dish with olive oil.
2. Cut all zucchinis lengthwise and then in segments.
3. In a non-stick skillet, add zucchini with ¼ cup water and cover for 2 minutes. Stir till water is completely evaporated or till zucchini is a little soft but not mushy.
4. Drain excess water and place the zucchini on baking sheet. Spread tomato sauce over them.
5. Top with Italian seasoning, garlic powder, salt and pepper and turkey pepperoni slices.
6. Put the baking sheet in oven and bake for 20 minutes.
7. Let it sit for 2 minutes and serve.

New York Style Paleo Pizza

Ingredients

Tomato sauce – 1 cup

Bacon strips – 1 cup

Mushroom – 1 cup (sliced)

Pepperoni slices – 12 (sliced)

Broccoli – 1 cup (chopped)

Olives – ½ cup (sliced)

Dried oregano – ½ tsp

Directions

1. Prepare crust by following the Paleo Pizza Crust recipe (mentioned in the start on the book).
2. Sauté bacon strips under crisp. Add pepperoni slices, mushrooms and broccoli. Pour in the tomato sauce and stir for one minute. Set aside.
3. After the crust is done, spread on the tomato sauce mixture.
4. Sprinkle with olives and oregano.
5. Bake for 15 minutes and serve warm.

Fresh Veggie Paleo Pizza

Ingredients

Basil – 2 tbsp

Garlic – 1 clove (minced)

Tomato sauce – 1 cup

Paprika – 1 tsp

Bell pepper – 1 (sliced)

Onion – 1 (sliced)

Zucchini – 1 (sliced)

Tomato – 1 (sliced)

Mushrooms – ½ cup (sliced)

Celery – 1 (sliced)

Olives – ½ cup (sliced)

Broccoli – ½ cup (chopped)

Egg plant – ½ cup (chopped)

Directions

1. Prepare crust by following the Paleo Pizza Crust recipe (mentioned in the start of the book).
2. Mix chopped basil and minced garlic with tomato sauce.
3. Spread this mixture over the crust when it is done.
4. Top with all the fresh veggies and sprinkle with paprika.
5. Bake for 10 minutes or till veggies are done.
6. Cut slices and serve.

Breakfast Bacon & Egg Pizza

Ingredients

Bacon strips – 1 cup

Tomato sauce – 1 cup

Eggs – 4

Olive oil – 2 tbsp

Onion – 1 (chopped)

Green bell pepper – 1 (chopped)

Salt and pepper – to taste

Red chili flakes – to taste

Directions

1. In a bowl mix bacon and tomato sauce. Add salt and pepper.
2. Make the pizza dough following the Paleo Pizza Crust recipe (mentioned in the start of the book).
3. Separate the dough in four small 6" pizza pans evenly. Spread the bacon sauce mixture on all the pans.
4. Bake for 15-20 minutes or till bacon is crisp.
5. Take out the pans and crack 1 egg in each of them. Add onions and bell peppers. Sprinkle olive oil, red chili flakes, salt and pepper over them.
6. Bake them again for 5-10 minutes or till the eggs are set.
7. Serve warm.

Final Words

Following a healthy Paleo diet does not mean you have to give up pizza. There are several ways you can make a perfectly healthy crust, top it with fresh veggies and meat of your choice. You will be surprised how many Paleo pizza options you have. These 50 Paleo Pizza recipes complied in this book are mouth-watering and delicious, that too without the extra calories you consume in a regular pizza.

What are you waiting for? Go on and try out these scrumptious healthy pizza recipes. Impress your friends and family with these healthy pizzas and add a bit of your own creativity as well.